Colon Cancer and Mental Health

Coping Strategies for Patients and Survivors

Dr. Gary A. Hudgins

Table of Content

Introduction

About this book

"Colon Cancer and Mental Health: Coping Strategies for Patients and Survivors" is a comprehensive guide that offers insights into the often-overlooked mental health challenges faced by those diagnosed with colon cancer. This book provides practical tips and strategies for coping with the emotional toll of colon cancer diagnosis and treatment.

Written by healthcare professionals, cancer survivors, and mental health experts, this book covers a range of topics including managing stress and coping with treatment, navigating relationships and support systems, dealing with work and financial concerns, self-care strategies for patients and survivors, and the role of mental health professionals in colon cancer care.

With a compassionate and understanding tone, "Colon Cancer and Mental Health" offers hope and inspiration to those facing the diagnosis and provides a valuable resource for family members and caregivers who are supporting their loved ones through this difficult time.

In this book, you'll learn about the emotional impact of colon cancer and discover coping strategies for dealing with fear, anxiety, and depression. You'll also find practical tips for managing stress and treatment side effects, maintaining healthy relationships, and navigating work and financial concerns.

The book also explores the benefits of self-care practices such as exercise, nutrition, mindfulness, and art therapy. Additionally, you'll discover the importance of seeking support from mental health professionals and learn how to find the right provider for your needs.

"Colon Cancer and Mental Health" is an empowering resource that offers a holistic approach to cancer care. It recognizes the importance of addressing mental health concerns in addition to physical symptoms and provides tools for promoting well-being throughout the cancer journey.

Whether you're a patient, survivor, or caregiver, this book will help you understand the impact of colon cancer on mental health and provide you with the tools you need to cope with the challenges that arise. With the insights and guidance offered in "Colon Cancer and Mental Health," you can prioritize your mental health and find hope and healing on your cancer journey.

The connection between colon cancer and mental health

The connection between colon cancer and mental health refers to the ways in which a diagnosis of colon cancer and its treatment can impact a person's emotional well-being.

When someone receives a diagnosis of cancer, it can be a life-altering event that can bring about a range of emotions such as shock, fear, and uncertainty. This can be especially true for colon cancer, as it is a disease that can be difficult to talk about due to its location and associated symptoms. The emotional impact of a diagnosis can also be compounded by the physical symptoms associated with colon cancer, such as changes in bowel habits, fatigue, and pain.

The treatment process for colon cancer can also have a significant impact on mental health. Surgery, chemotherapy, radiation therapy, and other treatments can be physically and emotionally challenging, and can lead to symptoms such as fatigue, nausea, and changes in mood or behavior.

In addition, colon cancer and its treatment can have a significant impact on a person's quality of life. For example, it may interfere with work and daily activities, and it can strain relationships with family and friends. This can create stress, which can exacerbate mental health concerns such as anxiety and depression.

In addition to addressing the emotional impact of colon cancer, it's important to recognize that mental health and physical health are interconnected. Studies have shown that mental health can have a significant impact on a person's physical health, and vice versa.

For example, stress and anxiety can weaken the immune system, making it more difficult for the body to fight off infections and illnesses, including cancer. Chronic stress has also been linked to inflammation, which can contribute to the development and progression of many chronic diseases, including colon cancer.

On the other hand, improving mental health can also have positive effects on physical health. For example, practicing stress-reduction techniques like mindfulness and meditation has been shown to reduce inflammation and improve immune function. Exercise and a healthy diet can also improve both physical and mental health.

By recognizing the connection between mental health and physical health, patients and caregivers can take a more holistic approach to cancer care. This includes addressing both physical and emotional needs, and seeking support to manage the associated challenges.

Acknowledging the connection between colon cancer and mental health is important because it allows patients and caregivers to recognize the emotional toll of the disease and seek support to manage the associated challenges. By addressing mental health concerns, patients can improve treatment outcomes and enhance their overall well-being. Seeking professional help, building a support network, and practicing self-care are all critical steps in addressing the mental health needs of those affected by colon cancer.

Overview of the book

Colon Cancer and Mental Health" is a comprehensive guide that explores the emotional impact of colon cancer and offers strategies for managing mental health concerns throughout the cancer journey. The book recognizes the interconnectedness of physical and mental health and provides insights into the ways in which colon cancer can impact a person's emotional well-being.

The book is divided into several sections, starting with an overview of colon cancer and its treatment, and then exploring the emotional challenges associated with the disease. The book also offers practical tips for managing stress, treatment side effects, and other challenges related to colon cancer, such as maintaining healthy relationships and navigating work and financial concerns.

The book emphasizes the importance of self-care practices such as exercise, nutrition, and mindfulness, and offers guidance on finding the right mental health support. Additionally, the book explores the role of complementary therapies such as art therapy and music therapy in promoting cmotional well-being.

Overall, "Colon Cancer and Mental Health" is a resource for patients, survivors, and caregivers who are seeking to better understand the emotional challenges associated with colon cancer and develop strategies for managing their mental health. The book offers practical advice, emotional support, and a holistic approach to cancer care, recognizing the importance of addressing mental health concerns in addition to physical symptoms.

Chapter 1

<u>The Emotional Impact of Colon Cancer</u>

The shock of diagnosis

The shock of diagnosis refers to the intense emotional response that many people experience when they receive a cancer diagnosis, including colon cancer. This response can be overwhelming and can include a range of emotions such as fear, disbelief, anger, and sadness. The shock of diagnosis is a normal and understandable reaction to a life-changing event such as a cancer diagnosis.

For colon cancer patients, the shock of diagnosis can be compounded by the discomfort and stigma associated with the disease, which can make it difficult for patients to share their diagnosis with others and seek support. Additionally, patients may feel overwhelmed by the need to make important decisions about their treatment options and care, which can further exacerbate the shock of diagnosis.

Managing the shock of diagnosis requires a multifaceted approach that addresses the emotional and physical aspects of the disease. Seeking support from loved ones, joining support groups, and connecting with mental health professionals can all be helpful in managing the emotional challenges of the disease. Additionally, patients may find it helpful to educate themselves about their diagnosis and treatment options, and to take an active role in their care.

It is important to note that the shock of diagnosis can impact patients and caregivers differently. Caregivers may also experience a range of emotions in response to a loved one's cancer diagnosis, including anxiety, guilt, and sadness. It can be challenging for caregivers to manage their emotions while also supporting their loved one, and it is important for them to seek support and self-care strategies as well.

In addition to the emotional impact of a cancer diagnosis, patients may experience physical symptoms related to the disease and its treatment, such as fatigue, pain, and changes in bowel habits. These symptoms can further exacerbate the shock of diagnosis and may make it difficult for patients to cope with their emotions. It is important for patients to communicate openly with their healthcare team about any physical symptoms they are experiencing, as addressing these symptoms can improve quality of life and reduce emotional distress.

By acknowledging the shock of diagnosis and seeking support, patients and caregivers can better manage the emotional challenges of the disease and move forward with their care.

Dealing with fear and anxiety

Dealing with fear and anxiety is a common challenge for people with colon cancer, as well as for their caregivers. The diagnosis of cancer can bring up a range of emotions, including fear, anxiety, and uncertainty about the future. Fear and anxiety can be further compounded by the physical symptoms associated with colon cancer, such as pain, fatigue, and changes in bowel habits. These symptoms can be distressing and can make it difficult for patients and caregivers to cope emotionally.

One of the most effective ways to manage fear and anxiety is to seek support. Support can come in many forms, such as talking to family members or friends, joining a support group, or connecting with a mental health professional. Support can provide patients and caregivers with a safe and supportive space to express their emotions and receive validation and understanding from others who have gone through a similar experience. Support can also help to reduce feelings of isolation and loneliness, which can be common for people with cancer.

In addition to seeking support, educating oneself about the disease and its treatment can be helpful in managing fear and anxiety. Learning about the disease can help to demystify it and provide patients and caregivers with a sense of control over their situation. Reliable sources of information include healthcare providers, reputable organizations like the American Cancer Society, and peer-reviewed medical journals.

Mind-body techniques can also be helpful in managing fear and anxiety. These techniques include practices like mindfulness meditation, deep breathing, and yoga. Mind-body techniques can help patients and caregivers relax, reduce stress, and manage difficult emotions.

In some cases, medications may be prescribed to help manage anxiety and other related symptoms. These medications can be prescribed by a healthcare provider and should be used in conjunction with other treatment strategies.

It is important to note that fear and anxiety can have physical manifestations, such as increased heart rate, sweating, and muscle tension. These physical symptoms can further exacerbate emotional distress and impact quality of life. For this reason, managing fear and anxiety is an important aspect of the overall care plan for people with colon cancer.

In addition to seeking support, education, and practicing mind-body techniques, there are other strategies that can be helpful in managing fear and anxiety. For example, setting achievable goals can help patients and caregivers feel a sense of accomplishment and control. Engaging in hobbies or activities that bring joy and relaxation can also be helpful in managing stress and anxiety.

It is important to recognize that fear and anxiety can ebb and flow throughout the cancer journey. It is normal for these emotions to resurface during times of uncertainty or during treatment, and patients and caregivers should be prepared to use the coping strategies that have worked for them in the past.

Ultimately, dealing with fear and anxiety is a normal and expected part of the colon cancer experience. Seeking support, educating oneself, practicing mind-body techniques, and using medications when necessary can all be effective strategies for managing these difficult emotions.

Coping with depression

Coping with depression is another common challenge for people with colon cancer, as well as for their caregivers. Depression is a mood disorder that can cause persistent feelings of sadness, hopelessness, and lack of interest or pleasure in activities. The diagnosis of cancer can be a major stressor that triggers or exacerbates symptoms of depression. In addition, the physical symptoms of colon cancer and its treatments, such as pain, fatigue, and changes in appetite, can also contribute to feelings of depression.

It is important to recognize the signs and symptoms of depression and seek help if needed. Symptoms of depression can include:

- Persistent feelings of sadness, emptiness, or hopelessness
- Loss of interest or pleasure in activities that were once enjoyable
- Changes in appetite and weight
- Sleep disturbances
- Fatigue or loss of energy
- Feelings of worthlessness or guilt
- Difficulty concentrating or making decisions
- Thoughts of suicide or self-harm

If you or someone you know is experiencing any of these symptoms, it is important to seek help from a healthcare provider or mental health professional.

Treatment for depression can include therapy, medication, or a combination of both. Therapy can provide patients and caregivers with a safe and supportive space to express their emotions and learn coping skills for managing depression. Medications, such as antidepressants, can help to alleviate symptoms of depression and improve overall mood.

In addition to therapy and medication, there are other strategies that can be helpful in managing depression. Regular exercise, healthy eating, and good sleep hygiene can all improve mood and overall well-being. Engaging in activities that bring joy and relaxation can also be helpful in managing symptoms of depression.

It's important to remember that coping with depression is not a sign of weakness, and seeking help is a sign of strength. Depression is a common and treatable condition, and getting the right support and treatment can help patients and caregivers feel better and improve their quality of life.

In the context of colon cancer, coping with depression can also involve addressing any concerns about the future, such as the possibility of recurrence or the impact of the disease on daily life. Therapy can provide patients and caregivers with tools to manage these worries and develop strategies for coping with uncertainty.

It's important to note that coping with depression is a process that can take time and effort. Patients and caregivers should be patient with themselves and each other, and recognize that healing takes time. With the right support and treatment, however, it is possible to manage depression and improve overall well-being.

In summary, coping with depression is a common challenge for people with colon cancer, as well as for their caregivers. It's important to recognize the signs and symptoms of depression, seek help from a healthcare provider or mental health professional, and use a combination of therapy, medication, and other coping strategies to manage the emotional challenges of the disease and improve overall quality of life.

The impact on self-esteem and body image

A diagnosis of colon cancer can have a significant impact on a person's self-esteem and body image. The physical changes that can occur as a result of the disease and its treatment, such as weight loss, hair loss, and scars, can be challenging for patients to cope with. In addition, some patients may experience changes in bowel function or other bodily functions that can affect their self-image and confidence.

As a result, it is common for patients with colon cancer to experience feelings of embarrassment, shame, or insecurity related to their appearance or bodily functions. These feelings can impact overall self-esteem and quality of life.

It is important for patients and caregivers to recognize that these feelings are normal and valid, and to seek support to help manage them. Support can come from healthcare providers, mental health professionals, and support groups.

Therapy can be helpful in addressing issues related to self-esteem and body image. A therapist can provide a safe and supportive space to explore these feelings and develop coping strategies for managing them. In addition, therapists can help patients and caregivers to identify and challenge negative thought patterns that may be contributing to low self-esteem.

Support groups can also be helpful for patients and caregivers dealing with issues related to self-esteem and body image. These groups can provide a sense of community and connection with others who are going through similar experiences. Support group members can share tips and strategies for managing physical changes and addressing negative self-talk.

In some cases, patients may also experience changes in sexual function as a result of colon cancer and its treatment. This can further impact self-esteem and body image, as well as strain intimate relationships. Healthcare providers and mental health professionals can provide support and resources to help patients and their partners navigate these challenges.

In addition, it's important for patients and caregivers to take care of their physical health, as this can have a positive impact on self-esteem and body image. Eating a healthy diet, getting regular exercise, and practicing self-care can all help patients feel better about themselves and their bodies.

Finally, it's important to remember that self-esteem and body image are complex issues that can be impacted by a range of factors beyond cancer. Patients and caregivers may benefit from exploring these issues in therapy, even after the cancer is in remission or cured.

Ultimately, coping with the impact of colon cancer on self-esteem and body image is an important aspect of the disease experience. By seeking support from healthcare providers, mental health professionals, and support groups, patients and caregivers can develop strategies for managing these challenges and improve their overall quality of life.

Finding meaning and purpose

Finding meaning and purpose can be a transformative experience for patients and caregivers dealing with colon cancer. It can help them to reframe their experience, find hope and motivation, and feel a greater sense of agency and control.

For some, finding meaning and purpose may involve exploring new avenues of personal growth or creative expression.

This can provide a sense of accomplishment and help patients to build resilience and confidence in their abilities.

For others, finding meaning and purpose may involve giving back to their community or helping others who are going through similar experiences. This can provide a sense of connection and purpose, and help patients and caregivers to feel that their experiences have value and meaning beyond themselves.

Therapy can be a helpful tool for patients and caregivers who are struggling to find meaning and purpose in their lives. A therapist can help them to explore their values, goals, and beliefs, and develop strategies for finding meaning and purpose in the face of illness.

In addition, support groups can be a valuable resource for patients and caregivers who are looking to connect with others who are going through similar experiences. These groups can provide a sense of community and support, as well as offer opportunities to share stories and insights about finding meaning and purpose.

Finding meaning and purpose can also help patients and caregivers to cope with the emotional and psychological impact of a colon cancer diagnosis. It can provide a sense of hope and positivity, which can help to counteract feelings of despair or hopelessness.

Moreover, finding meaning and purpose can help patients and caregivers to cultivate a sense of resilience in the face of challenges. By focusing on what is meaningful and important, patients and caregivers can build a sense of inner strength and purpose that can sustain them through difficult times.

One important aspect of finding meaning and purpose is cultivating a sense of gratitude. Despite the challenges of colon cancer, patients and caregivers can focus on what they are grateful for, whether it is the support of loved ones, access to quality healthcare, or the beauty of the natural world. By cultivating a sense of gratitude, patients and caregivers can shift their focus from what they have lost to what they still have, and find a sense of meaning and purpose in their lives.

Ultimately, finding meaning and purpose is an ongoing process that may require patience, self-compassion, and a willingness to explore new possibilities. By working with healthcare providers, mental health professionals, and support groups, patients and caregivers can develop the skills and strategies they need to cope with the challenges of colon cancer and find a sense of purpose and fulfillment in their lives.

Chapter 2

<u>Managing Stress and Coping</u>

<u>with Treatment</u>

The stress of treatment

Dealing with the stress of treatment can be overwhelming for patients and caregivers. In addition to managing the physical side effects of treatment, they may also be dealing with emotional and psychological stress, such as anxiety, depression, and uncertainty about the future.

One key strategy for coping with the stress of treatment is self-care. Patients and caregivers can prioritize activities that promote physical and emotional well-being, such as eating a healthy diet, getting enough sleep, engaging in regular exercise or physical activity, and practicing relaxation techniques such as meditation or deep breathing.

In addition, patients and caregivers can work with their healthcare team to manage treatment-related side effects, such as pain, nausea, fatigue, or digestive problems. This may involve adjusting medications, using complementary therapies such as massage or acupuncture, or seeking out additional support from mental health professionals or support groups.

Another important strategy is to seek out emotional support from loved ones or professionals. Patients and caregivers may benefit from talking openly about their fears and concerns, seeking counseling or therapy, or participating in support groups with other patients and caregivers who are going through similar experiences. This can help to reduce feelings of isolation and provide a sense of validation and support.

It is also important for patients and caregivers to maintain a sense of perspective and focus on the present moment. By staying mindful and focused on the here and now, patients and caregivers can reduce anxiety about the future and maintain a sense of hope and positivity.

One important aspect of coping with the stress of treatment is to stay informed and educated about the disease and its treatment. This can help patients and caregivers feel more in control and empowered in their healthcare decisions.

Patients can work with their healthcare providers to understand the goals and potential outcomes of treatment, and to make informed decisions about their care.

It is also important for patients and caregivers to be patient and compassionate with themselves. Coping with cancer and its treatment is a difficult process, and it is natural to experience a range of emotions and challenges. Patients and caregivers can give themselves permission to feel their emotions and to seek support when needed.

Finally, maintaining a sense of hope and positivity can be an important part of coping with the stress of treatment. This can involve finding meaning and purpose in the journey, connecting with others who have faced similar challenges, and focusing on the things that bring joy and fulfillment.

In the end, coping with the stress of treatment requires a multifaceted approach that addresses physical, emotional, and psychological needs. By taking care of themselves and seeking support from others, patients and caregivers can navigate the challenges of treatment and maintain a sense of hope and resilience.

Coping with treatment side effects

Side effects of colon cancer treatment can vary depending on the type of treatment used. For example, chemotherapy may cause nausea, fatigue, hair loss, and an increased risk of infection, while radiation therapy may cause skin irritation, fatigue, and digestive issues.

It is important for patients to work closely with their healthcare team to manage treatment side effects. This may involve adjusting medication dosages, trying different medications or therapies to alleviate side effects, or seeking out additional support from other healthcare providers, such as nutritionists or physical therapists.

In addition to medical treatments, patients may also benefit from complementary therapies to manage treatment side effects. For example, acupuncture or massage therapy may help alleviate nausea or pain, while yoga or meditation may help reduce stress and anxiety.

Patients should also take care of their physical health by eating a balanced diet, staying hydrated, getting enough sleep, and engaging in regular exercise or physical activity. This can help to manage treatment side effects and promote overall well-being.

Finally, it is important for patients to be aware of their own emotional needs and seek out support when needed. Coping with treatment side effects can be challenging, both physically and emotionally. Patients can seek out support from loved ones, mental health professionals, or support groups with other cancer patients.

Another important aspect of coping with treatment side effects is being proactive in managing symptoms. This can involve keeping track of symptoms and their severity, and communicating with healthcare providers about any changes or concerns. For example, if a patient is experiencing persistent nausea, they may need to adjust their diet or medication regimen to better manage this symptom.

Patients may also benefit from working with a healthcare provider or specialist who focuses on managing side effects. For example, a nutritionist can provide guidance on maintaining a healthy diet during treatment, while a physical therapist can help patients manage fatigue and maintain strength and flexibility.

In addition to seeking out medical and complementary treatments, patients can also take steps to promote their own emotional well-being. This may involve engaging in relaxation techniques such as deep breathing, visualization, or mindfulness meditation. Patients may also find it helpful to engage in activities that bring them joy and fulfillment, such as spending time with loved ones, pursuing hobbies, or volunteering in the community.

Ultimately, coping with treatment side effects requires a comprehensive and personalized approach that addresses each patient's unique needs and experiences. By working closely with their healthcare team, practicing self-care, and seeking out support, patients can manage treatment side effects and improve their overall quality of life.

The benefits of relaxation techniques

Relaxation techniques can provide numerous benefits for individuals dealing with the stress and challenges of colon cancer treatment. Here are a few key benefits of incorporating relaxation techniques into one's coping strategies:

1. Reduced stress and anxiety: Relaxation techniques such as deep breathing, meditation, and progressive muscle relaxation can help calm the mind and reduce feelings of stress and anxiety. This can help improve overall well-being and may even boost the immune system.
2. Improved sleep: Many relaxation techniques are designed to help quiet the mind and promote a sense of calm, which can help improve sleep quality. Getting adequate sleep is important for overall physical and emotional health, and can help individuals better manage the challenges of cancer treatment.

3. Reduced pain and discomfort: Relaxation techniques such as guided imagery or visualization can help individuals focus their attention away from pain or discomfort, which can help reduce its intensity or frequency. This can be especially helpful for individuals dealing with treatment-related pain or side effects.

4. Increased sense of control: Cancer treatment can be overwhelming and leave individuals feeling like they have lost control over their lives. Engaging in relaxation techniques can provide a sense of control and empowerment, as individuals take an active role in managing their own well-being.

5. Improved quality of life: By reducing stress and anxiety, improving sleep, and managing pain

or discomfort, relaxation techniques can help improve overall quality of life for individuals dealing with colon cancer.

6. Improved emotional well-being: Engaging in relaxation techniques can also help improve emotional well-being by providing a sense of calm and promoting feelings of positivity and relaxation. This can be especially important for individuals dealing with the emotional challenges of cancer treatment, such as depression or anxiety.

7. Reduced fatigue: Many individuals undergoing cancer treatment experience fatigue, which can be debilitating and impact quality of life. Relaxation techniques can help reduce fatigue by promoting

relaxation and improving sleep quality.

8. Reduced muscle tension: Relaxation techniques such as progressive muscle relaxation or guided imagery can help reduce muscle tension and improve overall physical relaxation. This can be especially helpful for individuals dealing with physical discomfort or pain related to cancer treatment.

9. Improved coping skills: Engaging in relaxation techniques can also help individuals develop better coping skills, which can be useful not only during cancer treatment but in other aspects of life as well. By learning to manage stress and anxiety, individuals may find that they are better able to cope with future challenges.

10. Increased overall well-being: By providing a sense of calm, promoting relaxation, and improving emotional and physical well-being, relaxation techniques can help improve overall quality of life for individuals dealing with colon cancer.

Strategies for managing stress and anxiety during treatment

Here are a few strategies for managing stress and anxiety during cancer treatment:

1. Mindfulness meditation: Mindfulness meditation involves focusing on the present moment

without judgment. This can help

reduce anxiety by allowing

individuals to let go of worries about

the future or regrets about the past.

Mindfulness meditation can be

practiced in a variety of ways, such

as through guided meditation

sessions or simply by focusing on

the breath.

2. Relaxation techniques: As discussed

earlier, relaxation techniques such as

deep breathing, progressive muscle

relaxation, and guided imagery can

help reduce stress and anxiety by promoting relaxation.

3. Exercise: Regular exercise can help reduce stress and anxiety by releasing endorphins, which are natural mood-boosters. Even light exercise such as walking or gentle yoga can be helpful.

4. Support groups: Support groups can be a valuable resource for individuals dealing with colon cancer, providing a space to connect with others going through similar

experiences and share coping
strategies.

5. Therapy: Working with a therapist
can help individuals develop coping
strategies for managing stress and
anxiety related to cancer treatment.
Cognitive-behavioral therapy (CBT)
is a type of therapy that has been
shown to be particularly effective for
individuals dealing with
cancer-related stress and anxiety.

6. Self-care: Engaging in activities that
bring joy or relaxation can be an
important part of managing stress

and anxiety. This might include reading, taking a bath, or spending time in nature.

7. Medication: In some cases, medication may be necessary to manage stress and anxiety related to cancer treatment. Individuals should discuss medication options with their healthcare team to determine if this is an appropriate option for them.

8. Dietary changes: Making changes to the diet can also be helpful for managing stress and anxiety during cancer treatment. For example,

avoiding caffeine and sugar, eating a balanced diet rich in fruits and vegetables, and staying hydrated can all help reduce stress and improve mood.

9. Art therapy: Art therapy involves using creative expression, such as drawing, painting, or sculpting, as a way to process emotions and reduce stress. This can be a helpful tool for individuals who find it difficult to express their emotions verbally.

10. Massage therapy: Massage therapy can help reduce stress and

promote relaxation by reducing muscle tension and improving circulation. It can also be a helpful tool for managing treatment-related symptoms such as pain or nausea.

11.   Acupuncture: Acupuncture involves the insertion of thin needles into specific points on the body to promote relaxation and reduce stress. It has been shown to be effective for managing cancer-related symptoms such as pain and fatigue.

12.   Pet therapy: Spending time with animals can be a helpful way to

reduce stress and improve mood. Pet therapy involves interacting with trained animals in a therapeutic setting, and has been shown to be effective for individuals dealing with cancer-related stress and anxiety.

It's important to remember that everyone's experience with colon cancer is unique, and what works for one person may not work for another. It's important to explore different strategies and find the ones that work best for you. With the support of a healthcare team, loved ones, and a variety of coping strategies, it's possible to manage stress and anxiety and maintain a sense of well-being during colon cancer treatment.

Chapter 3

<u>Navigating Relationships and Support Systems</u>

Talking to family and friends about your diagnosis

When someone is diagnosed with colon cancer, it can be a difficult and emotional experience, and it's natural to want to turn to family and friends for support. However, talking to loved ones about a cancer diagnosis can also be challenging, and it's important to consider how to approach these conversations in a way that feels comfortable and supportive.

One important consideration is to be clear about your own needs and preferences. For example, some people may prefer to keep their diagnosis private, while others may want to share their experience with a wider circle of family and friends. It can also be helpful to think about who you want to tell first, and how you want to communicate the news (in person, by phone, or through a letter or email).

Another consideration is how to manage the emotions that can come up when talking to loved ones about cancer. For example, family and friends may feel scared, sad, or overwhelmed by the news, and it can be helpful to acknowledge and validate these feelings. It can also be helpful to set clear boundaries around what kind of support you need, and to be open to receiving help from loved ones.

Finally, it's important to remember that everyone's experience with cancer is different, and it's normal to feel a range of emotions throughout the journey. By being open and honest with loved ones, and by seeking support from a healthcare team and other resources, it's possible to navigate the challenges of a colon cancer diagnosis with resilience and grace.

In addition to considering your own needs and preferences when talking to family and friends about your diagnosis, it can also be helpful to have a support system in place. This may include close friends or family members who can provide emotional support, as well as healthcare professionals who can offer medical guidance and treatment options.

It's also important to remember that loved ones may have their own reactions and emotions to your diagnosis, and it can be helpful to provide resources and support for them as well. This may include connecting them with support groups or counseling services, or simply providing them with information about colon cancer and its treatment.

Another important consideration when talking to family and friends about your diagnosis is how to manage the practical aspects of cancer treatment. For example, you may need help with transportation to medical appointments, or assistance with household chores during periods of fatigue or recovery.

Ultimately, talking to family and friends about a colon cancer diagnosis is a deeply personal decision, and there is no right or wrong way to approach these conversations. However, by being open and honest with loved ones, and by seeking support from healthcare professionals and other resources, it's possible to navigate the challenges of a colon cancer diagnosis with compassion and resilience.

Maintaining healthy relationships during treatment

Maintaining healthy relationships with loved ones during colon cancer treatment can be a challenge, but it is essential for emotional and physical well-being. Here are some strategies for maintaining healthy relationships during colon cancer treatment:

1. Communicate openly: It's important to communicate openly with your

loved ones about your feelings and needs during treatment. Be honest about how you're feeling physically and emotionally, and let them know how they can best support you.

2. Set boundaries: Setting clear boundaries can help prevent misunderstandings and conflicts. Let your loved ones know when you need space or when you're feeling overwhelmed.

3. Practice self-care: Taking care of yourself during treatment is crucial for maintaining healthy relationships. Make time for activities that bring you joy and relaxation, and prioritize your physical and emotional well-being.

4. Seek support: Joining a support group or seeking counseling can be helpful in navigating the emotional

challenges of cancer treatment. This can also help alleviate the burden on loved ones who may be struggling to provide emotional support.

5. Express gratitude: Expressing gratitude and appreciation for the support of loved ones can help strengthen relationships and foster positivity during a challenging time.

6. Be patient: Understand that loved ones may not always know how to support you in the best way, and it may take time for them to adjust to your diagnosis and treatment. Be patient with them and try to communicate your needs in a gentle and compassionate way.

7. Be open to help: Accepting help from loved ones can be difficult, but it's important to remember that they want to support you in any way they

can. Allow them to help with tasks such as cooking, cleaning, or running errands if it eases your burden.

8. Include loved ones in treatment: Inviting loved ones to accompany you to doctor's appointments or treatments can help them feel involved and provide a sense of support. This can also be an opportunity to educate them about your diagnosis and treatment.

9. Don't be afraid to ask for space: While it's important to maintain relationships during treatment, it's also essential to prioritize your own needs. Don't be afraid to ask for space or time alone when you need it.

10. Be aware of your emotions: Cancer treatment can be emotionally draining, and it's normal to

experience a range of emotions. However, it's important to be aware of how your emotions may be impacting your relationships with loved ones. Try to communicate your feelings in a healthy and constructive way.

By practicing patience, being open to help, and including loved ones in treatment, it's possible to maintain healthy relationships during colon cancer treatment. Remember that the journey may be challenging, but with support from loved ones, you can overcome this obstacle together.

Finding support groups and resources

Finding support groups and resources is an important step in coping with colon cancer. Support groups can provide emotional and practical support, as well as a safe space to share experiences and connect with others who are going through similar challenges.

Here are some ways to find support groups and resources:

1. Ask your healthcare team: Your healthcare team can provide information about support groups and resources that may be available in your area.
2. Search online: There are many online support groups and resources

available for those with colon cancer. Some popular options include the Colon Cancer Alliance and the American Cancer Society.

3. Join social media groups: Many social media platforms have groups dedicated to colon cancer support. These groups can provide a sense of community and support, as well as opportunities to connect with others who are going through similar experiences.

4. Attend local events: Local events such as fundraisers and awareness walks can provide an opportunity to connect with others in your community who have been affected by colon cancer.

5. Consider professional counseling: A mental health professional can provide individualized support and

counseling to help you cope with the emotional challenges of colon cancer.

In addition to support groups, there are many other resources available to those with colon cancer. These resources can help you better understand your diagnosis, treatment options, and ways to cope with the emotional challenges of living with cancer.

Some common resources include:

1. Educational materials: There are many books, websites, and other educational materials available that provide information about colon cancer, treatment options, and strategies for coping.
2. Patient advocacy organizations: Patient advocacy organizations, such

as the Colon Cancer Alliance and Fight Colorectal Cancer, can provide information, resources, and advocacy on behalf of colon cancer patients and their families.

3. Financial assistance programs: Some organizations offer financial assistance to help with the costs of treatment, such as transportation, lodging, and medication.

4. Nutrition counseling: Proper nutrition is an important part of cancer treatment, and many healthcare providers offer nutrition counseling to help patients maintain a healthy diet during treatment.

5. Complementary therapies: Some patients find that complementary therapies such as acupuncture, massage, and meditation can help them cope with the physical and

emotional side effects of cancer treatment.

It's important to remember that every patient's needs and experiences are unique, and what works for one person may not work for another. By exploring different resources and finding what works best for you, you can build a support network that helps you navigate the challenges of living with colon cancer.

Addressing caregiver stress and burnout

Caregivers play a critical role in supporting individuals with colon cancer. However, the demands of caregiving can be overwhelming, leading to stress and burnout. It's important for caregivers to prioritize their own well-being to avoid burnout and provide the best possible care.

Here are some strategies that caregivers can use to manage stress and prevent burnout:

1. Seek support: Caregiving can be isolating, so it's important for caregivers to seek out support from family, friends, and healthcare professionals. This can include talking with a therapist, attending a

support group, or reaching out to a social worker.

2. Take breaks: Caregivers need to take time for themselves to recharge and prevent burnout. This can include taking a short walk, reading a book, or engaging in a favorite hobby.

3. Prioritize self-care: Caregivers should make sure to prioritize their own physical and emotional well-being. This can include eating a healthy diet, getting enough sleep, and engaging in regular exercise.

4. Accept help: It's okay for caregivers to accept help from others. This can include delegating tasks to family members or hiring a professional caregiver.

5. Manage expectations: Caregivers should manage their expectations for themselves and the person they are caring for. It's important to recognize that caring for someone with colon cancer can be challenging, and that it's okay to ask for help.

It's also important for caregivers to have open and honest communication with the person they are caring for. This includes discussing their preferences for care, treatment options, and any concerns or fears they may have.

Caregivers should also be aware of the signs of depression, anxiety, and other mental health concerns in both themselves and the person they are caring for. It's important to seek help from a healthcare professional if these issues arise.

In addition, caregivers should be prepared to navigate the healthcare system and advocate for their loved one. This can include scheduling appointments, communicating with healthcare providers, and coordinating care with other members of the healthcare team.

Finally, caregivers should be aware of the financial and logistical challenges of caring for someone with colon cancer. This may include navigating insurance coverage, arranging transportation to appointments, and managing medication and treatment costs.

By addressing caregiver stress and burnout, caregivers can provide the best possible care and support for their loved one with colon cancer, while also taking care of their own well-being.

Chapter 4

<u>Dealing with Work and Financial Concerns</u>

Communicating with your employer

When you receive a colon cancer diagnosis, you may need to take time off work to receive treatment or recover. It's important to communicate with your employer about your diagnosis and treatment plan so that they can make appropriate accommodations for you.

This may include taking time off work for medical appointments or treatment, working from home, or adjusting your work schedule. It's important to be honest and transparent with your employer about your needs and limitations, while also being respectful of their needs as a business.

The Americans with Disabilities Act (ADA) and Family and Medical Leave Act (FMLA) may provide legal protections and accommodations for people with cancer in the workplace. It's important to familiarize yourself with these laws and your rights as an employee.

It can be helpful to have a conversation with your employer early on in the process to establish a plan for managing your work responsibilities while also taking care of your health. This can help reduce stress and anxiety for both you and your employer.

In addition to communicating with your employer, it can also be helpful to connect with a human resources representative or benefits coordinator at your workplace to discuss any available resources or support. This may include information on healthcare benefits, disability insurance, and employee assistance programs (EAPs) that can provide emotional support and counseling for you and your family.

It's important to keep in mind that the stress of cancer treatment can take a toll on your physical and emotional health, as well as your ability to work. It may be necessary to take a leave of absence or reduce your work hours during this time. However, with the right support and accommodations, many people are able to successfully manage their cancer treatment and work responsibilities.

If you're struggling to communicate with your employer or are experiencing discrimination or unfair treatment in the workplace due to your cancer diagnosis, it may be helpful to consult with a lawyer or advocate who specializes in cancer-related workplace issues. There are also many cancer support organizations that offer resources and guidance on navigating employment and financial issues during cancer treatment.

Overall, addressing the impact of a cancer diagnosis on your work life is an important aspect of managing your overall well-being and quality of life during treatment. By communicating openly with your employer, accessing available resources, and advocating for your rights as an employee, you can help ensure that you receive the support you need to navigate this challenging time.

Navigating insurance and financial concerns

Navigating insurance and financial concerns is an important aspect of managing a cancer diagnosis. Cancer treatment can be expensive, and understanding your insurance coverage and financial options can help alleviate some of the stress and anxiety associated with these costs.

One important step is to review your health insurance coverage and understand your out-of-pocket costs, such as deductibles, copays, and coinsurance. It may be helpful to speak with a representative from your insurance company or a financial counselor to clarify any questions or concerns you have about your coverage.

It's also important to explore any financial assistance programs that may be available to you. Many hospitals and cancer centers offer financial assistance programs for patients in need, and there are also national organizations that provide financial support for cancer patients and their families.

In addition, it's important to consider the potential impact of cancer treatment on your work and finances. Depending on your treatment plan and the nature of your work, you may need to take time off from work or reduce your hours. This can have a significant impact on your income and financial stability, so it may be helpful to explore options such as short-term disability or other leave policies.

To navigate insurance and financial concerns, it is important to be proactive and informed. One way to do this is to keep track of all medical bills and expenses related to your cancer treatment. This can help you identify any errors or discrepancies in billing, and can also be useful for tax purposes or when applying for financial assistance.

Another important step is to be an informed consumer when it comes to healthcare. This means researching and comparing treatment options and costs, and asking questions about the necessity and cost-effectiveness of different treatments. It may also be helpful to explore options such as clinical trials, which can provide access to cutting-edge treatments at reduced or no cost.

In addition, it's important to be an advocate for yourself when it comes to insurance and financial concerns. This may involve negotiating with your insurance company or medical providers to reduce costs, or seeking help from a patient advocacy organization or legal aid service.

Finally, it's important to take care of your mental and emotional well-being during this process. Coping with the financial stress of cancer treatment can be overwhelming, and it's important to seek support and resources to manage these challenges. This may include seeking counseling or support from a social worker or mental health professional, or connecting with support groups or online communities for cancer patients and their families.

Coping with work-related stress

Coping with work-related stress is an important aspect of managing cancer and its treatment. Cancer diagnosis and treatment can often have a significant impact on your ability to work, both physically and mentally. It is important to communicate with your employer about your needs and limitations and explore options for workplace accommodations.

One of the first steps is to inform your employer about your diagnosis and any treatment plans. This can be difficult, but it is important to have an open and honest dialogue with your employer about your situation. This will help your employer understand your needs and limitations, and can also help them identify ways to support you during this time.

Depending on the nature of your job, you may need to consider making changes to your work schedule or duties to accommodate treatment schedules or side effects. It may be necessary to take time off work for treatments or appointments, and it is important to know your rights and options for taking leave under the Family and Medical Leave Act (FMLA) or other employment laws.

Your employer may also offer workplace accommodations, such as flexible work schedules, telecommuting, or ergonomic adjustments to your workspace. You may also be eligible for disability benefits or other forms of financial assistance to help offset the costs of cancer treatment.

It's important to prioritize self-care and stress management during this time. This may involve finding ways to manage stress at work, such as taking breaks, delegating tasks, or practicing mindfulness or relaxation techniques. It may also involve seeking support from coworkers, friends, or a mental health professional.

In summary, coping with work-related stress involves open communication with your employer, exploring workplace accommodations, knowing your rights and options for leave and financial assistance, and prioritizing self-care and stress management.

Chapter 5

<u>Self-Care Strategies for Patients and Survivors</u>

Prioritizing self-care during and after treatment

Prioritizing self-care during and after treatment is an essential aspect of cancer survivorship. Cancer and its treatment can take a toll on a person's physical and emotional well-being, leading to increased stress, fatigue, and a diminished quality of life. It is crucial for survivors to take care of themselves both during and after treatment to help mitigate the impact of the disease and its treatment.

Self-care can take many different forms, including physical activity, good nutrition, adequate rest, and stress-reduction techniques. Exercise can help improve overall health and reduce the risk of recurrence, while proper nutrition can help support the immune system and aid in healing. Adequate rest is also essential for recovery, as fatigue is a common side effect of cancer treatment.

Stress-reduction techniques such as mindfulness meditation, yoga, or tai chi can help reduce stress levels and improve overall well-being. Additionally, survivors may benefit from support groups or counseling services to help them cope with the emotional impact of the disease and its treatment.

It is also important for survivors to stay engaged in their healthcare, including follow-up appointments and recommended screenings. Regular check-ups and screenings can help detect any potential health concerns early, which can improve the chances of successful treatment and long-term survival.

Overall, prioritizing self-care during and after cancer treatment is crucial for survivors' well-being and long-term health. By taking care of themselves physically, emotionally, and spiritually, survivors can improve their quality of life and increase their chances of long-term survival.

The benefits of exercise and nutrition

The benefits of exercise and nutrition refer to the positive effects that engaging in regular physical activity and consuming a balanced diet can have on individuals diagnosed with colon cancer. Studies have shown that exercise can help reduce fatigue, improve overall quality of life, and reduce the risk of cancer recurrence. Proper nutrition, including a diet high in fruits, vegetables, whole grains, and lean protein, can also have a positive impact on cancer outcomes.

Exercise has been shown to improve physical and emotional well-being in cancer patients, with benefits including increased energy levels, improved sleep, reduced anxiety and depression, and increased muscle strength and endurance. It is also thought to help reduce the risk of colon cancer recurrence and other chronic diseases.

Nutrition is also important for cancer patients, as a healthy diet can help reduce inflammation and oxidative stress in the body, which can contribute to cancer development and progression. Eating a diet rich in fruits, vegetables, whole grains, and lean protein can also help maintain a healthy body weight, which is important for overall health and cancer outcomes.

Regular exercise and a balanced diet can have many benefits for those with colon cancer. Exercise has been shown to improve physical function, reduce fatigue, and improve mood and overall quality of life. In addition, a healthy diet can help boost the immune system and improve digestion, which can be especially important during and after treatment.

Mindfulness and meditation practices

Mindfulness and meditation practices are techniques that involve focusing one's attention on the present moment and accepting it without judgment. These practices are often used to reduce stress, increase emotional well-being, and promote relaxation. In the context of coping with colon cancer, mindfulness and meditation can be helpful in reducing anxiety, depression, and other negative emotions that may arise during treatment.

Mindfulness practices may involve techniques such as deep breathing, body scans, and visualization exercises. Meditation practices may involve sitting or lying down in a quiet space and focusing on a specific object or mantra. These practices have been shown to reduce stress hormones, lower blood pressure, and improve overall physical and emotional well-being.

In addition to reducing stress and anxiety, mindfulness and meditation practices have been found to have a range of other benefits for cancer patients. For example, these practices have been shown to improve immune function, which can help patients to better fight off infections and other illnesses during treatment.

Mindfulness and meditation can also help patients to better manage pain and discomfort associated with cancer and its treatment. By focusing on their breath and learning to observe their thoughts and emotions without judgment, patients can develop a greater sense of control over their physical sensations and reduce the impact of pain on their daily lives.

Another benefit of mindfulness and meditation practices is that they can improve cognitive function, including memory and attention span. This can be particularly important for cancer patients who may experience "chemo brain" or other cognitive impairments as a result of treatment.

Overall, mindfulness and meditation practices can be valuable tools for coping with the emotional and physical challenges of colon cancer. These practices can help patients to develop greater resilience, reduce stress, and improve overall quality of life during and after treatment.

Art therapy and other creative outlets

Art therapy and other creative outlets refer to using various forms of art to express oneself and explore emotions, thoughts, and feelings. Art therapy is a form of psychotherapy that involves using art materials and creative processes to improve a person's physical, mental, and emotional well-being.

In the context of coping with colon cancer, art therapy and other creative outlets can provide a safe and expressive way to explore and process emotions related to the cancer diagnosis and treatment. It can also be a way to find joy and relaxation during a difficult time.

Some examples of creative outlets for coping with colon cancer include:

- Painting or drawing
- Writing poetry or journaling
- Playing music or listening to music
- Taking photographs or making videos
- Making crafts or scrapbooking
- Participating in theater or acting

Art therapy and other creative outlets can be powerful tools in coping with the emotional and psychological effects of colon cancer. Expressive arts, such as drawing, painting, and sculpting, can provide a nonverbal outlet for emotions, allowing individuals to communicate and process feelings that may be difficult to express in words. It can also serve as a form of relaxation and stress reduction, promoting a sense of calm and wellbeing.

Creative expression can also serve as a form of distraction from the physical and emotional symptoms of cancer and treatment, allowing individuals to focus on something positive and fulfilling. Additionally, participating in creative activities can foster a sense of accomplishment and pride, boosting self-esteem and confidence.

Art therapy may be facilitated by a trained therapist, but individuals can also engage in creative activities on their own or with the support of loved ones. Other forms of creative expression, such as music, dance, and writing, can also offer similar benefits and provide additional avenues for self-expression and coping.

Chapter 6

<u>The Role of Mental Health Professionals in Colon Cancer Care</u>

The Role of Mental Health Professionals in Colon Cancer Care refers to the importance of seeking support from mental health professionals, such as psychologists or therapists, during and after colon cancer treatment. These professionals can help patients and their families cope with the emotional and psychological challenges that come with a cancer diagnosis, such as anxiety, depression, and post-traumatic stress disorder.

Mental health professionals can also assist patients in managing treatment-related symptoms, such as pain and fatigue, by teaching relaxation techniques, providing cognitive-behavioral therapy, and offering support groups. They can also help patients adjust to changes in their lifestyle and body image and provide guidance in addressing relationship issues and other concerns related to cancer.

In addition, mental health professionals can help patients navigate the healthcare system and advocate for themselves, which is especially important when dealing with complex medical issues and insurance-related concerns. By addressing the mental and emotional aspects of cancer care, mental health professionals can improve patients' quality of life and overall well-being.

The benefits of therapy and counseling

When facing a serious health condition such as colon cancer, it's common for individuals to experience a range of emotional and psychological distress. Therapy and counseling can offer a space for individuals to process their thoughts and emotions, learn coping strategies, and develop a plan for managing their mental health during and after treatment.

One of the key benefits of therapy and counseling is the opportunity to work with a trained mental health professional who can offer guidance and support in navigating the emotional challenges of a cancer diagnosis. Therapists and counselors can help individuals identify and work through fears and anxieties related to treatment, manage symptoms of depression and anxiety, and improve communication with loved ones.

Additionally, therapy and counseling can help individuals develop effective coping skills that can improve their overall quality of life. This may include techniques such as mindfulness, cognitive-behavioral therapy (CBT), and relaxation techniques. These skills can not only help individuals manage the stress and anxiety associated with cancer treatment but also improve their ability to cope with other life challenges.

It's important to note that therapy and counseling are not one-size-fits-all solutions, and it may take some time to find the right therapist and approach for each individual's unique needs. However, with the support of a mental health professional, individuals can improve their emotional well-being and better manage the challenges of colon cancer.

Therapy and counseling can provide significant benefits for individuals who are coping with colon cancer. These mental health professionals are trained to help individuals process their emotions, address their fears and anxieties, and develop coping strategies to manage the challenges of cancer treatment.

Therapy can take many different forms, including individual counseling, family therapy, and group therapy. Individual counseling allows the person to work one-on-one with a therapist, exploring their feelings and developing personalized coping strategies. Family therapy can be particularly helpful for individuals who are dealing with the impact of cancer on their relationships with loved ones. Group therapy can provide a supportive environment where individuals can connect with others who are going through similar experiences.

In addition to traditional talk therapy, there are also several other types of therapy that may be helpful for individuals with colon cancer. For example, cognitive-behavioral therapy (CBT) can help individuals change negative thought patterns and behaviors that may be contributing to their stress and anxiety. Mindfulness-based stress reduction (MBSR) can help individuals cultivate a greater sense of calm and focus, even in the midst of difficult circumstances.

Ultimately, the goal of therapy and counseling is to help individuals with colon cancer improve their quality of life and find meaning and purpose in their experience. With the help of mental health professionals, individuals can learn to manage their stress and anxiety, cope with treatment side effects, and build stronger relationships with loved ones.

Types of mental health professionals

There are several types of mental health professionals who can provide support and care for individuals coping with colon cancer. These may include:

1. Psychologists: Psychologists are trained to diagnose and treat mental health disorders and provide counseling and therapy to individuals and families.

2. Psychiatrists: Psychiatrists are medical doctors who specialize in mental health disorders and can prescribe medication to manage symptoms.

3. Social workers: Social workers can provide counseling and connect individuals with resources and support services in their community.

4. Licensed Professional Counselors (LPC): LPCs provide therapy and counseling to individuals, couples, and families to address mental health concerns and improve overall well-being.

5. Behavioral health specialists: These professionals work in cancer centers and hospitals to provide mental health support to individuals and families affected by cancer.

6. Spiritual counselors: Some individuals may find comfort in speaking with a spiritual counselor,

such as a chaplain or religious leader, who can offer emotional support and guidance during difficult times.

7. Oncology nurses: Oncology nurses are specially trained to care for individuals with cancer. They can provide emotional support and help individuals manage the physical side effects of cancer treatment.

8. Palliative care specialists: Palliative care specialists are trained to provide care and support to individuals with serious illnesses, including cancer. They can help manage symptoms and improve quality of life.

9. Licensed marriage and family therapists (LMFTs): LMFTs have a

master's degree in marriage and family therapy and are licensed to provide therapy and counseling to couples and families. They can help families cope with the emotional impact of colon cancer and provide support during treatment and recovery.

10.   Licensed clinical social workers (LCSWs): LCSWs have a master's degree in social work and are licensed to provide therapy and counseling. They may also connect individuals with community resources and support services.

It is important for individuals to find a mental health professional who is experienced in working with cancer patients and understands the unique challenges and stressors associated with cancer diagnosis and treatment.

Finding the right mental health provider for you

Finding the right mental health provider is an important step in addressing the emotional and psychological impact of a colon cancer diagnosis. There are different types of mental health professionals who can provide support and care during this time, including psychologists, social workers, licensed professional counselors, and psychiatrists.

When looking for a mental health provider, it's important to consider factors such as their experience and expertise, their approach to treatment, and their availability. Some individuals may prefer to see a therapist who has experience working with cancer patients, while others may prioritize finding someone who specializes in cognitive-behavioral therapy or another evidence-based treatment approach.

It's also important to consider practical factors such as location, insurance coverage, and scheduling availability. Some individuals may prefer to see a therapist who offers remote or virtual sessions, while others may prioritize finding a provider who is located nearby.

When it comes to finding the right mental health provider for you, there are several things to consider. First and foremost, it's essential to choose someone who specializes in working with cancer patients and understands the unique challenges that come with a cancer diagnosis.

Other factors to consider include their qualifications, experience, and approach to treatment. Some mental health professionals may use cognitive-behavioral therapy, while others may use psychoanalytic or humanistic approaches. It's crucial to choose a provider who aligns with your values and preferences.

It's also essential to consider practical factors such as insurance coverage, location, and availability. You may want to check with your insurance provider to see which providers are covered under your plan, and you may need to consider the logistics of scheduling appointments around your cancer treatments and other obligations.

Ultimately, finding the right mental health provider is about finding someone you feel comfortable with and trust to help you navigate the emotional challenges of cancer. Don't be afraid to ask questions, seek referrals, and take the time to find the right fit for you.

Conclusion

In conclusion, this book aimed to provide guidance and support for those who have been diagnosed with colon cancer and are struggling with mental health challenges. Throughout the pages, we have explored the emotional impact of diagnosis, coping strategies for dealing with fear, anxiety, and depression, and the importance of self-care and seeking professional help.

As we reflect on the journey of this book, we are reminded of the resilience and strength of those who have faced a cancer diagnosis. It is our hope that the information and tools provided in these pages have been helpful and empowering for readers.

While the road ahead may still be challenging, it is important to remember that there is always hope and support available. We encourage readers to continue seeking out resources and support, whether it be from loved ones, mental health professionals, or community organizations.

As we close this chapter, we hope that this book has provided not only practical guidance but also a sense of comfort and community for those who may be struggling with mental health challenges related to colon cancer.

Final thoughts and resources for support

In conclusion, a colon cancer diagnosis can be a challenging and overwhelming experience that can take a significant toll on a person's mental health. However, it is essential to remember that mental health support and resources are available to help individuals cope with the emotional and psychological aspects of their diagnosis and treatment.

Throughout this book, we have explored various strategies and resources that can aid in managing the emotional impact of colon cancer, from coping with the shock of diagnosis to maintaining healthy relationships and prioritizing self-care during and after treatment. We have discussed the role of mental health professionals in colon cancer care and highlighted the benefits of therapy, counseling, and other mental health practices.

Remember that you are not alone, and seeking support is a sign of strength. If you or a loved one is struggling with the emotional impact of colon cancer, reach out to a mental health professional or support group for guidance and assistance.

Below are some additional resources that may be helpful in managing the emotional impact of colon cancer:

- The American Cancer Society's Cancer Survivors Network provides an online community for cancer survivors and caregivers to connect and share their experiences.
- The Colon Cancer Alliance offers support groups, educational resources, and advocacy initiatives

for individuals and families affected by colon cancer.

- The National Cancer Institute's Cancer Information Service provides free, confidential information and support for cancer patients and their families.

- The National Alliance on Mental Illness (NAMI) offers resources and support for individuals with mental illness and their families.

Remember, taking care of your mental health is just as important as taking care of your physical health. With the right support and resources, you can navigate the emotional challenges of colon cancer and find hope and healing on your journey.

www.ingramcontent.com/pod-product-compliance
Lightning Source LLC
Chambersburg PA
CBHW070846250726
48662CB00003B/1388

9 798391 020127